Supplements for
FIBROMYALGIA

DR. JOE M. ELROD

WOODLAND PUBLISHING
Pleasant Grove, Utah

CONTENTS

Introduction

Fibromyalgia is a common clinical syndrome of generalized musculoskeletal pain, stiffness, and chronic aching at specific points of the body. The condition is considered primary when it is not associated with a systemic cause such as trauma, cancer, thyroid disease, and pathologies of rheumatic arthritis or connective tissues. It is now recognized as one of the most common rheumatic complaints in North America and has been the cause for 10 to 30 percent of all rheumatology consultations (Bennett, 1989). Although research from the early part of this century identified inflammation in muscles as the main cause of the condition, research done in the past 50 years has produced substantial evidence that inflammation does not play a significant role in fibromyalgia. The most important recent discovery concerning fibromyalgia is that the causes are such that intervention is possible and the symptoms can be reversed.

What Causes Fibromyalgia?

Rather than arthritis of the joints, fibromyalgia is actually a form of muscular and "soft tissue" rheumatism. Rheumatism refers to the pain and stiffness associated with arthritis and related disorders of the joints, muscles, and bones. Fibromyalgia mainly affects muscles and their attachments to bones, especially in the areas of muscle/tendon junctions (Bennett, 1989).

A single, exact cause of fibromyalgia is not known, but experts attribute the onset of the condition to a variety of factors. Because these factors have been identified, an effective treatment regimen can be identified. The following events or conditions commonly contribute to the onset of fibromyalgia:

- traumatic emotional experience
- stress and/or depression
- magnesium, phosphate, substrate, and oxygen deficiencies

- biological disruption of energy production
- chronic fatigue
- low levels of growth hormone
- disruption of deep sleep

Symptoms of Fibromyalgia

Fibromyalgia is referred to as a syndrome because it is a set of signs and symptoms that occur together. (A sign is what the physician or health professional finds on examination; a symptom is what the person reports to the health care professional or the doctor.) The major symptoms of fibromyalgia are listed below:

- tenderness of at least 11 of 18 specific anatomical sites
- pain
- chronic aching
- stiffness
- sleep disorders
- fatigue
- stress/anxiety
- depression
- vitamin and mineral deficiencies

Most patients with fibromyalgia syndrome state that they literally ache all over. They describe their muscles as feeling like they have been pulled, torn, or overworked, sometimes twitching and at other times burning. The severity of symptoms will fluctuate tremendously from one person to the next. Fibromyalgia syndrome sometimes resembles a post-viral state, which is one of the reasons some experts and researchers in the field believe that fibromyalgia syndrome and chronic fatigue syndrome are one and the same (Goldenberg, 1990). According to Wolfe (1993), the only thing that differentiates between the two is the degree of pain. Brief discussions of these symptoms follow.

PAIN AND STIFFNESS

The pain associated with fibromyalgia syndrome is the most prominent symptom of the condition. Patients describe the pain as deep, burning, throbbing, and stabbing. The pain is generally felt throughout the body, although it starts in one region such as the neck and shoulders, and then seems to spread over time to other parts of the body. The pain will often vary, depending on the time of day, activity level, the weather, sleep patterns, and interruptions in lifestyle. Most fibromyalgia patients report that some degree of pain is consistently present.

SLEEP DISORDERS AND FATIGUE

During sleep we usually have periods when we stop moving and go into a deep, very restful, recharging sleep (level 4). Unfortunately, in fibromyalgia, the pain of the muscles and connective tissue makes it impossible to lie in one position for an extended period of time. As a result the patient is continually brought back into light sleep. Fibromyalgia patients simply do not experience the deep stages of sleep that allow for complete rest. Even when they sleep for eight hours each night they can awaken tired each morning (May, 1993). Scientific studies (Campbell, 1983) indicate that most people with fibromyalgia have an abnormal sleep pattern marked by interruptions in their deep sleep. This type of disorder is one of the more devastating symptoms of fibromyalgia syndrome

The fatigue associated with fibromyalgia has been described as "brain fatigue," in which people feel totally drained of energy. The fatigue symptom can be mild in some and incapacitating in others. Ninety percent of those with fibromyalgia describe moderate or severe fatigue similar to the exhaustion experienced with the flu. Very often fatigue is more of a problem than pain. Many patients state that they feel as if their arms are tied to concrete blocks and they have great difficulty concentrating.

STRESS AND TRAUMA

The exact initial trigger for symptoms in fibromyalgia such as faulty pain filters and disrupted energy production and sleep cycles is largely unknown. However, the more prominent theory appears to be severe stress coupled with emotionally traumatic experiences, especially over extended periods of time. A 1994 study revealed such findings and supported a peripheral origin for fibromyalgia pain (Russell, 1996). Crofford (1994) and Moldofsky (1995) have identified similar neuroendocrine abnormalities in other studies which help to continue to form the basis of the etiology of fibromyalgia.

Another theory currently being evaluated as a possible cause of fibromyalgia is the body's response to stress and trauma. Researchers are trying to determine if the autonomic nervous system works properly under such conditions. Long periods of undue stress and emotional disruption appear to be the underlying cause of energy compound deficiencies. Over long periods, trauma interrupts the natural physiological process of ATP (energy) production. Along with prolonged stress and trauma, poor diet, lack of exercise, and lack of the proper nutrients and supplements (vitamins, minerals, and antioxidants) will begin to weaken the immune system to the point that the body will yield to the onset of fibromyalgia. Fortunately, the fibromyalgia sufferer has control over many of these factors and can use that control to overcome fibromyalgia symptoms.

Vitamin and Mineral Deficiencies

Thiamin (B1), riboflavin (B2), and pyridoxine (B6) are essential for electron transport in the respiratory system. To become biologically active, all three vitamins require a magnesium-dependent phosphate transferring action. When there is a magnesium deficiency, the body's energy production process breaks down. Magnesium is one of the key ingredients of the formula and it has been found that almost all fibromyalgia patients have a magnesium deficiency. Most migraine headache victims will also demonstrate a magnesium deficiency.

Some current research now indicates that fibromyalgia sufferers are deficient in certain compounds, including the magnesium required for the production of energy. The presence of magnesium, substrate oxygen, and phosphates are essential for energy production. Concentrations at very high levels are required for healthy cellular respiration and production of biological energy. And deficiencies in these substances can seriously impede the Krebs cycle (human energy cycle), causing a reduction of the ability of the body to utilize oxygen for muscle energy. Current research has confirmed that a deficiency of the above factors can very clearly lead to the symptoms of fatigue and depression in the fibromyalgia victims.

MAGNESIUM AND MALIC ACID— A HELPFUL COMBINATION

Aluminum has been identified as a toxic metal leading to major metabolic disturbances, so researchers have carefully studied means of eliminating it from the body's vital organs. They have discovered that proper amounts of magnesium, along with supplemental malic acid, can act as a most potent aluminum detoxifier. Together these substances are especially effective at decreasing aluminum toxicity in the vital organs of the body, especially the brain. Malic acid is effective because it has been shown to significantly increase the fecal and urinary secretion of aluminum, reducing the concentration of the metal found in the internal organs, tissues, and the brain (Weintraub, 1997).

MANGANESE—A CRITICAL SUPPLEMENT

Recent studies have investigated the link between chronic fatigue syndrome and fibromyalgia syndrome, specifically why fatigue is one of the most prominent features in both syndromes. It may have something to do with manganese-dependent neuroendocrine changes, especially along the hypothalamic-pituitary-thyroid axis. The hypothalaums produces thyrotropin-releasing hormones (TRH). TRH stimulates the pituitary gland to produce thyroid-stimulating hormones (TSH) which in turn stimulate thyroid production of thyroxin.

This is critical simply because thyroxin regulates the metabolic rate. Since fatigue is one of the primary conditions of both fibromyalgia and chronic fatigue victims, an underactive metabolism due to secondary hypothyroidism fits very nicely into the hypothesis. Manganese directly influences the metabolic rate through its involvement in this hypothalamic-pituitary-thyroid axis. Therefore, it may be a helpful trace mineral supplement for both fibromyalgia and chronic fatigue victims. It would make good sense for those with fibromyalgia to supplement with magnesium, malic acid, and manganese for the production of energy, for aluminum detoxification, to enhance metabolism, and return to general health and well-being.

Curing Fibromyalgia

Many doctors believe that the chronic problems of musculoskeletal pain and fatigue are incurable—the patient is told only that the pain is somewhat manageable through the use of drugs and therapy. But the truth is that many sufferers have returned to vibrant, productive, and healthy lives by making healthy changes in diet and lifestyle. Natural treatments are a key factor in making these changes. Supplemental vitamins, minerals and natural preparations can do much to reverse the symptoms of fibromyalgia, and many are backed by scientific evidence. The remainder of this booklet will discuss the most effective alternative treatments and the most recent research in reversing fibromyalgia.

Natural Remedies and Supplements—An Overview

More and more physicians are becoming interested in alternative and natural treatments that utilize the products of Mother Nature. This is primarily a result of the positive data underscoring their effectiveness in helping people regain and maintain their health and vitality. At the same time, the conventional physician may not be that knowledgeable about natural treatments because of limited time. The average physician is hard pressed just to keep up on all the new drugs, let alone study all the breakthroughs on herbs, vitamins, minerals, supplements and nutritional treatments.

People with fibromyalgia and other chronic conditions should use caution when self-treating without the guidance of a physician or health professional who is well trained in nutrition. There are so many products and so much information available that it is easy to be confused about what to use and how to use it. However, with proper guidance, you can be successful in returning to vibrant health and an active lifestyle. The following is a list and description of the minerals, vitamins, herbs, and supplements that may be helpful for fibromyalgia and other systemic conditions.

Minerals Are Crucial

Much research has been done regarding the importance of minerals in the body and their function in healthy development. Minerals are absolutely the most important of all the body's nutrients. Even though the body needs only small amounts of many minerals, they need to be supplied on a daily basis to maintain and regulate necessary body functions. It is necessary to supplement the diet with minerals and other nutrients. Minerals are key because vitamins, amino acids, enzymes, fats, and carbohydrates all require minerals for their activity. Without minerals, they cannot be absorbed and utilized.

More and more people are suffering from mineral deficiencies as minerals continue to disappear from our soils and food supply. This appears to be one of the major problems of the fibromyalgia sufferer. After long periods of undue stress and emotional disruption there is almost always a deficiency of some of the minerals, especially magnesium. When there is a deficiency of minerals, the result is a nutritional imbalance that can lead to a disruption of sleep patterns, concentration, and the ability to interact normally (Weintraub, 1997). Growing evidence supports the fact that stress and anxiety over long periods of time result in mineral imbalances and this appears to be one of the primary factors that promotes the onset of fibromyalgia.

The following is a list of the important minerals and their nutritional value for the fibromyalgia sufferer and others with chronic conditions.

MAGNESIUM

This important mineral assists in the absorption of potassium, calcium, phosphorus, sodium, B-complex vitamins, as well as vitamins C and E. Magnesium is also a major regulator of cellular activity, including the maintenance of DNA and RNA, and it is considered an anti-stress mineral. For this reason magnesium has a calming effect and is effective when taken before bedtime. Magnesium is an essential part of the enzyme system but is poorly assimilated by the body, so it should be taken daily by the fibromyalgia sufferer. A chocolate craving is sometimes indicative of a magnesium deficiency and deficiencies are very common in times of stress, malabsorption, diarrhea, diabetes, and kidney disease. Some of the other symptoms of deficiency are weakness, depression, apprehension, irritability in the nerves and muscles, nausea, vomiting, sensitivity to noise, muscle cramps and insomnia.

In one study, Abraham, et al. (1992) demonstrated that significant reductions in pain/tenderness severity could be achieved during extended treatment with high doses of magnesium and malic acid. No limiting factors were found. Other researchers have found that fibromyalgia patients do indeed have significantly lower red blood cell magnesium levels compared to reference laboratory and osteoarthritis controls (Romano, 1997). Low tissue levels of magnesium in fibromyalgia were confirmed by Clauw (1994) who also showed that low muscular magnesium levels correlated with low pain tolerance. Magnesium supplementation has beneficial impacts on fatigue and pain.

CALCIUM

Calcium is critically essential because it is the most abundant mineral in the body. Most of the calcium in the body is located in the bones and the teeth. This mineral is necessary for the transmission of nerve signals and is important for the smooth functioning of the heart muscles and muscular movements of the intestines. It is very important for good health, especially for anyone who has a poor diet, suffers from malabsorption, or gets little sunshine. Calcium should be balanced with magnesium for proper nerve function and for a healthy body. Calcium, magnesium, and zinc all have a calming effect in the body and are very effective if taken before bedtime to help relax muscles and promote sleep. Vitamins A, C, D and phosphorus are also essential for the efficient functioning of calcium. Some of the symptoms of a calcium deficiency are tingling of the lips, fingers and feet, leg numbness, muscle cramps, and sensitivity to noise. (*Note:* Do not take antacids to make up for calcium deficiency.)

POTASSIUM

Potassium is responsible for normal heart and muscle function, normal transmission of nerve impulses, and normal growth. It works with sodium to regulate the flow of nutrients in and out of the cells and also helps to stimulate the kidneys and keep the adrenals healthy. It is also involved in the maintenance of heart rhythm and is vital in stimulating nerve impulses which cause muscle contraction. The symptoms of a potassium deficiency include muscle twitches, weakness and soreness, erratic and/or rapid heartbeats, fatigue, glucose intolerance, nervousness, high cholesterol, and insomnia.

CHROMIUM

Chromium is essential for the synthesis of fatty acids and the metabolism of blood sugars for energy. It is also known for increasing the efficiency of insulin in carbohydrate metabolism. Symptoms of a deficiency include weight loss, glucose intolerance, and psychological confusion.

SELENIUM

Selenium is considered an aid to other nutrients, especially vitamin E. It is considered a very powerful antioxidant and needed for immune function, cell membrane integrity, and for DNA metabolism. Selenium is another mineral considered very important for systemic conditions as it protects the body from the toxicity of drugs and heavy metals such as aluminum, cadmium, and mercury.

ZINC

Zinc is a vital component of enzymes in the brain that repair cells. It is very important for hearing, vision, taste, and helps to form skin, hair, and nails. Zinc also assists with the absorption of vitamins in the body and is essential for the many enzymes involved in digestion and metabolism. Vitamin A must be present for zinc to be properly absorbed by the body. Symptoms of a deficiency include depression, distorted taste sensation, diarrhea, brittle nails and hair, hair loss, fatigue, and memory loss.

MANGANESE

Manganese is found in many enzymes in the body and assists in the utilization of glucose. It also aids in reproduction and normal functioning of the central nervous system. Manganese is also vital for proper brain function, muscles, nerves and is very important for energy production. Some of the symptoms of a deficiency are nausea, dizziness, muscle coordination problems, strained knees, loss of hearing, slow growth of hair and nails, and low cholesterol.

PHOSPHORUS

Phosphorus and calcium work together and are found mainly in the bones and teeth. Phosphorus levels can be decreased by drinking too much soda pop, a lack of vitamin D, and stress. Phosphorus is essential for fibromyalgia sufferers because it helps to produce energy as it aids in the oxidation of carbohydrates. Some of the symptoms of a phosphorus deficiency are a loss of appetite, irregular breathing, nervous disorders, and insomnia.

IODINE

The body requires very little iodine, but this trace mineral is essential for the thyroid hormone thyroxine. When supported by iodine, the thyroid gland helps to facilitate energy production. A malfunctioning thyroid can, of course, cause symptoms of fatigue and lethargy. Other symptoms of iodine deficiency are swollen fingers and toes, dry hair, cold hands and feet, and irritability.

IRON

Iron is a mineral that everyone is very familiar with, yet many people suffer a deficiency in their nutritional programs. Iron is not easily absorbed by the body and requires an adequate amount of hydrochloric acid for proper assimilation. Vitamins C and E are also necessary if iron is to be utilized efficiently. Iron is known as the anti-anemia mineral because of its assistance in the oxygenation of cells and combining with protein to form hemoglobin.

Essential Vitamins

A significant number of people with fibromyalgia and other systemic conditions are suffering from vitamin deficiencies. Vitamins are complex organic substances necessary for life and good health. They are constantly used in the body and must be replaced daily. We obtain vitamins from the food we eat, from herbs, and from supplements. Vitamins are necessary for the body to utilize other nutrients. They contribute to breaking down fats, carbohydrates, and protein into usable forms. Vitamins should normally be taken before meals in order for proper absorption to take place. The following information on vitamins can benefit those with fibromyalgia and other systemic conditions:

VITAMIN A

Remember that vitamin A is a fat-soluble vitamin that can be toxic within the body if taken in large quantities. However, beta carotene is nontoxic and is converted to vitamin A in the body on an as-needed basis. This is why one can take up to 25,000 I.U. of beta carotene on a daily basis and not build up a toxic effect. This vitamin helps maintain and repair muscle tissue, treats skin problems, fights infection, and aids in the growth and maintenance of healthy bones, skin, teeth, and gums. Some good sources of vitamin A are yellow and green vegetables, eggs, milk, liver, fish liver oils, carrots, apricots, and sweet potatoes. Some symptoms of a vitamin A deficiency include dry hair, itchy and burning eyes, sinus trouble, and fatigue.

VITAMIN C (ASCORBIC ACID)

Vitamin C is a water-soluble vitamin that is essential to the body. It helps prevent infection by increasing the activity of white blood cells and assists in destroying viruses and bacteria. It also performs as a powerful antioxidant and is considered an antistress vitamin. Vitamin C is essential for healing and the synthesis of neurotransmitters in the brain and, when combined with bioflavonoids, also assists with adrenal and immune functions. It helps in the formation of collagen which is essential for good skin, bones, teeth, and growth in children.

The following conditions usually call for an increase in vitamin C: infections, fevers, injuries, excessive physical activity, anemia, and cortisone use. In one study, 26 patients with viral hepatitis took a vitamin C supplement daily for several weeks. Researchers concluded that vitamin C "exerts a remarkable immuno-modulating action." In patients with nasal irritation and congestion, vitamin C reduced symptoms in three-fourths of the patients (Null, 1993). Excellent sources of vitamin C include citrus fruits, cantaloupe, vegetables, broccoli, cauliflower, and red and green peppers. Some herbs that are good vitamin C sources are hawthorn berries, passionflower, olive oil, ginseng, and horsetail.

VITAMIN E (TOCOPHEROL)

One of the tremendous values of vitamin E for fibromyalgia sufferers is that it assists them in calming down and relaxing. Selenium increases the effectiveness of vitamin E and it is activated by vitamin A. It helps control the unsaturated fats in the body and is thought to reduce cholesterol, helps to normalize brain function, and protects glands during stress.

Studies looking at the results of elevated levels of vitamin E showed enhanced antibody response and improved white blood cell activity and immune response (Weiner, 1986). Vitamin E is also considered one of the powerful antioxidants and is needed for cholesterol metabolism, blood clotting, lung metabolism, muscle and nerve maintenance, and body cleansing. Some good sources of vitamin E are peanuts, vegetable oils, lettuce, wheat germs, whole grains, spinach, corn, and egg yolks. The herb kelp is plentiful in vitamin E.

B-COMPLEX VITAMINS

Fibromyalgia patients need more B vitamins since they are under a great deal of stress and B vitamins assist in the calming process and good mental health. They are also vital in the production of serotonin, a chemical in the body that influences calming behavior. When B vitamins are deficient due to inadequate nutrition or increased demand, it can significantly contribute to the lack of an ability to handle stress. B-complex vitamins work together to calm the nervous system and support correct brain function as well as to improve concentration and memory. Much care should be taken when taking the B vitamins as too much vitamin B6 is capable of causing a folic acid deficiency.

VITAMIN B1 (THIAMINE)

Vitamin B1 is necessary for digestion, blood cell metabolism, muscle metabolism, pain inhibition, and energy. Cellular magnesium abnormalities have been shown in studies to be associated with faulty vitamin B1 metabolism (Eisinger, 1994). B1 is a water soluble vitamin and needed in only small amounts on a daily basis. Some good sources of B1 are rice bran, wheat germ, oatmeal, whole wheat, sunflower seeds, brewer's yeast, and peanuts. Herbs that contain vitamin B1 are gotu kola, kelp, peppermint, slippery elm, and ginseng.

VITAMIN B2 (RIBOFLAVIN)

Vitamin B2 is necessary for antibody formation, red blood cell formation, cell respiration, fat and carbohydrate metabolism. B2 is also water soluble and must be replaced on a daily basis. It is also essential for proper enzyme formation, normal growth, and tissue formation. Some good sources of vitamin B2 are wild rice, liver, fish, white beans, sesame seeds, wheat germ, and red peppers. A few of the herbs containing B2 are gotu kola, kelp, peppermint, and ginseng.

VITAMIN B3 (NIACINAMIDE)

Vitamin B3 assists the body in producing insulin, female and male hormones, and thyroxine. B3 is also needed for circulation, acid production, and histamine activation. Some good sources of vitamin B3 are white meat, avocados, whole wheat, prunes, liver, and fish. Symptoms of a B3 deficiency are hypoglycemia, memory loss, irritability, confusion, diarrhea, ringing in the ears, depression, and insomnia.

VITAMIN B6 (PYRIDOXINE)

Vitamin B6 is helpful in converting fats and proteins into energy and in the production of red blood cells. It is also essential for proper chemical balance in the body. B6 is especially helpful to the fibromyalgia sufferer who is experiencing excessive stress. Symptoms of a B6 deficiency include irritability, nervousness, depression, muscle weakness, pain, headaches, PMS, and stiff joints.

VITAMIN B12 (COBALAMIN)

Vitamin B12 is essential for iron absorption, for the metabolism of fat, protein, and carbohydrates, for the formulation of blood cells, and for the long life of cells. A recent study also supports the use of B12 to combat fatigue. It was found that all fibromyalgia and chronic fatigue syndrome patients tested were found to have elevated levels of a substance called homocysteine in their central nervous systems. Homocysteine has been identified as a high risk factor in cardiovascular disease and high homocysteine levels have been correlated with both high levels of fatigue and low levels of vitamin B12 (Regland, 1997). Thus B12 supplementation would be beneficial in lowering homocysteine levels to fight fatigue and decrease chances of cardiovascular disease.

A strict vegetarian will need to supplement with vitamin B12. Some symptoms of a B12 deficiency include headaches, memory loss, dizziness, paranoia, muscle weakness, fatigue, and depression.

BIOTIN

Biotin is especially needed if you are under excessive stress, experiencing malabsorption, or have a poor nutrition program. Biotin aids in the metabolism of protein, fat, and carbohydrates, the production of fatty acids, and cell growth. Some of the symptoms of a biotin deficiency are muscle pain, nausea, anemia, fatigue, high cholesterol, and depression.

PANTOTHENIC ACID

Pantothenic acid is needed for the normal functioning of muscle tissue and protects membranes from infection. It is also essential for energy conversion, blood stimulation, and detoxification. Individuals under excessive stress and with poor diets need pantothenic acid to assist in normal body functioning. Symptoms of a deficiency include digestive problems, muscle pain, fatigue, depression, irritability, and insomnia. Pantothenic acid is vital for the fibromyalgia sufferer due to the above facts.

PARA AMINOBENZOIC ACID (PABA)

PABA assists in facilitating protein metabolism, promoting growth, and blood cell formation. Some of the symptoms of a PABA deficiency are depression, fatigue, irritability, nervousness, constipation, and, eventually, arthritis.

BIOFLAVONOIDS

Bioflavonoids work together with vitamin C to strengthen connective tissue and capillaries. Bioflavonoids are also essential in assisting the body to utilize most of the other nutrients. Good sources of bioflavonoids are spinach, cherries, rosehips, citrus fruits, apricots, blackberries, and grapes. Herbs that contain bioflavonoids are paprika and rosehips.

Herbal Supplements

Mother Nature provides herbs that have been used by mankind as healing agents since the dawn of history. In ancient times people were not aware that all the chemical elements contained in the leaves, root, bark, fruits, and flowers of herbs are the same chemicals that make up the human body. Modern technology has substantiated the use of herbal medicines and has proven why they have been used successfully for so long. Herbs contain various biochemical constituents—hormones, enzymes, vitamins, minerals, essential fatty acids, chlorophyll, fiber, and many other important elements. Herbs provide the body with what it needs to boost the immune system and to aid the body in healing itself.

Herbs are different from drugs in that they almost always contain elements in the amounts that nature intended. Herbalists believe that the natural approach of using herbs can add health and vigor to the body because herbs provide a broad array of catalysts which work together synergistically and harmoniously, resulting in the complete healing of the body in most cases.

Drugs made synthetically from plants are no longer in their natural form. As a result, people often find that these drugs cause more harm than good because of side effects. In contrast, herbs are natural, safe and do not build up in the body, producing side effects. There seem to be herbs that are of value to every system of the body. Still, herbs need to be used with wisdom and knowledge. They should not be used or mixed with other medications unless directed by a physician. The following is a list of some of the herbs and natural nutrients that may be of benefit to those with fibromyalgia and other systemic conditions:

RED CLOVER

Red clover is a natural blood purifier and builder and is normally used in its liquid form. It is used to give the body energy and to protect and strengthen the immune system. This herb is high in vitamin A and is an excellent choice in any tea-blend as it is usually more effective when complemented with other herbs. Some of the herbs complementary to red clover are prickly ash bark, echinacea, cascara bark, rosemary, and buckthorn bark.

Research has indicated that red clover contains some antibiotic properties that are beneficial against bacteria. This herb has been used for treating bronchitis, cancer, nervous conditions, and removing toxins from the body. It is invaluable to the fibromyalgia sufferer because it is high in selenium, which is very important in the nutritional regimen, and because it also contains manganese, sodium, calcium, copper, and magnesium. Red clover contains the B-complex vitamins and vitamin C as well, necessary for boosting the immune system and disease prevention.

PASSIONFLOWER

This herb has properties that are helpful for the nerves and circulation. Passionflower works well in formulas designed to treat insomnia and also works effectively in formulas designed to combat nervous tension, anxiety, stress, restlessness, and nervous headaches. Passionflower is helpful for fevers and is one of the more effective herbs for the nervous system.

VALERIAN

Valerian is probably the herb most widely used for anxiety and nervous tension. It is used as a natural sedative to improve the quality of sleep, relieve insomnia, and to combat depression. Valerian contains essential oils and alkaloids which reportedly combine to produce the calming, sedative effect. One study found that hyperactive individuals using valerian were able to concentrate for longer periods of time (Mowrey, 1993). Considered a nervine herb, valerian is used as a safe non-narcotic herbal sedative, and has also been used for after-pains in childbirth, heart palpitations, muscle spasms, and arthritis. Valerian is rich in calcium, which accounts for its ability to strengthen the spine, nerves, and brain. It is also high in magnesium, which works with calcium for healthy bones and the nervous system. It also contains high levels of selenium and manganese, good for strengthening the immune system, as well as containing zinc and vitamins A and C.

CHAMOMILE

Chamomile possesses relaxing properties that prove to be very effective in promoting relaxation and inducing sleep. It also promotes digestion and assists in assimilating nutrients from food, thereby enhancing metabolism and the utilization of energy. Ancient Egyptians used chamomile for its healing properties. Recent animals studies have proven chamomile to have antihistaminic effects along with anti-ulcer and antibacterial properties. The herb is useful for cleansing the liver, increasing mental alertness, promoting natural hormones, and for revitalizing the texture of skin and hair.

Chamomile is high in calcium and magnesium, two minerals that strengthen the nervous system, promote restful sleep, and improve the strength of the immune system. It also contains vitamins A, C, F, and B-complex, making it effective for the nervous system. Selenium and zinc, significant for the immune system, are also found in chamomile. Finally, the herb contains tryptophan, the component that allows it to work as a sedative and promote sleep.

PAU D'ARCO

Pau d'arco is reported to be a natural blood cleanser and builder. It also possesses antibiotic properties which aid in destroying viral infections in the body. It helps combat cancer and has been used to strengthen the body, increase energy, and strengthen the immune system.

GINSENG

Ginseng is one of the oldest and most beneficial herbs in the world. Research has shown that the roots are effective against bronchitis and heart disease. Ginseng has also been found to reduce blood cholesterol, improve brain function and memory, increase physical stamina, stimulate the endocrine glands, strengthen the central nervous system, and build the immune system.

Ginseng has been rated as the most potent of herbs because it supports so many body functions. It benefits the heart and circulation, normalizes blood pressure, and prevents arteriosclerosis. It is also used to help protect the body against radiation and as an antidote to drugs and toxic chemicals. Ginseng contains vitamin A and vitamin E, the component essential for a healthy heart and circulatory system. It also contains the B vitamins thiamine, riboflavin, B12, and niacin, all necessary for maintaining healthy nerves, hair, skin, eyes, and muscle tone. The minerals magnesium, iron, calcium, potassium, and manganese are also found in ginseng.

GOLDENSEAL

Goldenseal assists in boosting a sluggish glandular system and promoting hormone production. The herb is a very powerful nutrient that goes directly into the blood stream and assists in regulating liver function. Goldenseal is reported to act as a natural form of insulin by providing the body with nutrients necessary to produce its own insulin. This aids metabolism and energy production and makes goldenseal a very effective nutrient for fibromyalgia. It is also reported to act as a natural antibiotic to stop infections. Berberine, a key compound found in goldenseal, has been found to stimulate and boost the activity of macrophages that work to destroy invading bacteria, viruses, fungi and even tumor cells (Sack, 1982).

Goldenseal contains two alkaloids, hydrastine and hydrastinine, that have strong astringent and antiseptic effects on mucus membranes. The antibiotic properties of goldenseal are largely due to its alkaloid content, which has also been found to be effective against organisms such as staphylococcus, streptococcus, salmonella, and *Candida albicans*. Goldenseal is a very powerful immune booster. This herb contains vitamins A, C, E, F, and B-complex. It also contains potassium, phosphorus, iron, calcium, zinc, and manganese.

GOTU KOLA

Gotu kola is said to be a valuable treatment for depression by helping with mental fatigue and memory loss. Naturalists recommend gotu kola for rejuvenating the nervous system. It is sometimes referred to as "brain food" because of its ability to energize brain function. It is also used to increase circulation, neutralize blood toxins, help balance hormones, and relax the nerves. Gotu kola is rich in magnesium and also contains vitamins A, C, and K which protect the lungs from disease and the immune system against diseases. Vitamin K is necessary for blood clotting and in healing colitis. Gotu kola is a good source of manganese, niacin, zinc, calcium, sodium, and vitamins B1 and B2.

ALOE VERA

Although the aloe vera plant looks like a cactus, it is actually a member of the lily family. Aloe vera is known to promote healing when used externally, and it has been used effectively for treating radiation burns. Also vera is known to help increase movement in the intestines, promote menstruation, relieve constipation, and aid in digestion. In this way it works to aid the body in eliminating toxins. Another benefit of aloe is that it can be used to help with inflammation and ulcers. It also cleans, soothes, and relieves pain. It contains salicylic acid and magnesium which function together as an analgesic.

Aloe vera is high in vitamin C and selenium, two powerful antioxidants that help prevent and cure diseases. The results of a study done at the Tokyo Women's Medical College corroborated other findings that aloe vera is an immune enhancer. The study determined that lectins found in the aloe gel may help to stimulate response by increasing the production of lymphocytes known to kill bacteria (Foster, 1997). It also contains vitamins A and B-complex, phosphorus, magnesium, potassium, niacin, manganese, and zinc.

ECHINACEA

Echinacea is a powerful nutrient that stimulates the body's immune response and increases its ability to resist infection. It also assists in the production of white blood cells and is helpful as a blood purifier. Echinacea is considered a natural antibiotic. Extracts of the root have been found to contain interferon-like properties. Interferon is produced naturally in the body to prevent viral infections and has been known to fight chemical toxic poisoning in the body.

Echinacea contains vitamin C, which helps to promote healing and fights infections. Calcium and vitamin E are also found in this powerful herb, along with iodine that assists the thyroid gland in regulating metabolism, mental development, and energy production. It also contains potassium for muscle contraction, kidney function, and nerve function. The sulfur content of echinacea helps to dissolve acids in the body and improve circulation.

GRIFFONIA SIMPLICIFOLIA AND 5-HTP

The high prevalence of migraines among fibromyalgia sufferers suggests a common ground between fibromyalgia and migraines. Migraines are characterized by a defect in the serotonergic and adrenergic systems. A parallel dramatic failure of serotonergic systems and a defect of adrenergic transmission has been shown to also affect fibromyalgia sufferers. Enhancing serotonergic analgesia while increasing adrenergically mediated analgesia seems to be an important tool in fibromyalgia, and the administration of 5-hydroxytryptophan (5-HTP) significantly improved fibromyalgia. *Griffonia simplicifolia* is a natural source of 5-HTP. All the clinical variables (number of tender points, anxiety, pain intensity, quality of sleep, fatigue) showed a significant improvement when patients were given 5-HTP during extended treatment periods (Puttini, 1992).

ST JOHN'S WORT

Numerous studies on St. John's wort extracts involving depressed patients have been published in the last 20 years. In Germany, St. John's wort extracts are among the most widely prescribed antidepressants as well as the best selling, non-prescription antidepressant in the country. St John's wort extracts have consistently matched the antidepressant efficacy of synthetic antidepressants such as amitriptyline, imipramine, and maprotiline without side effects. Researchers observed beneficial effects within two weeks.

Seasonal affective disorder (SAD) is a subgroup of major depression. St. John's wort extracts, light therapy, and specific antidepressants have been shown to be beneficial. When bright light therapy combined with St. John's wort extract was compared to St. John's wort extract alone, there was no significant difference—indicating that the benefit was coming from the extract itself. St. John's wort extract was well tolerated and was recommended as a potentially efficient therapy in patients with SAD (Kasper, 1997).

KAVA

Another herbal extract that has been used for its calming effects on people with anxiety disorders is kava-kava, which in some cases is recommended over synthetic psychopharmacological agents (Laux, 1997). Three randomized placebo-controlled double-blind trials on anxiety disorders have recently been completed. In each clinical study, treatment demonstrated a high level of efficacy of kava extract associated with very good tolerance of the preparation. A good multidisciplinary overview of kava-kava is available (Singh, 1992).

BOSWELLIA SERRATA

Boswellia serrata is a traditional Ayurvedic treatment for joint pain and inflammation. In ancient times this material was known as frankinscence (Kirtikar 1935). *Boswellia serrata* has been found to have slow-acting, long term anti-inflammatory affects (Majeed, 1996). Mechanistically, *Boswellia serrata* appears to function as a natural inhibitor of leukotriene biosynthesis.

SLIPPERY ELM

Slippery elm is a demulcent which buffers against irritations and inflammations of the mucous membranes. A very powerful nutrient for fibromyalgia sufferers, it also promotes the activity of the adrenal glands and is a nutritious herb for both internal and external healing. It has been used primarily to treat stomach and intestinal ulcers, gastrointestinal problems, digestion acidity, and to lubricate the bowels. Slippery elm is also a blood builder and a supporter of the cardiovascular system. It is equal to oatmeal in vitamin and mineral content. The herb contains vitamins A, K, F, and P, all important in building and toning the lungs, stomach, and colon. Minerals contained in slippery elm are selenium, copper, zinc, iron, calcium, phosphorus, and potassium.

ROSEMARY

Rosemary is of great benefit in replacing aspirin for the treatment of headaches. This unique herb assists in combating stress and improving memory. It is high in calcium and is considered of benefit to the entire nervous system.

Other Supplements

GLUCOSAMINE SULFATE

Glucosamine is the key substance that determines how many proteoglycan (water-holding) molecules are formed in cartilage. It has been found very effective for improvement in arthritic conditions (and fibromyalgia is often called a soft-tissue arthritis). In a study conducted by the Vulvodynia Project, glucosamine was used to effectively reduce sensitivity and pain in soft tissue areas of fibromyalgia patients.

The use of glucosamine and and cartilage hydrolysates in the nutritional treatment of arthritic conditions has been well documented by Dr. Luke Bucchi (1995). Research also shows that glucosamine accelerates the repair of tissue injuries (Prudden, 1970). These soft tissue effects are in addition to the documented benefits of glucosamine and cartilage hydrolysates on joint function and pain reduction. Glucosamine improves inflammatory conditions as well as acting as a free-radical scavenger.

CHONDROITIN SULFATE

Chondroitin sulfates are naturally occurring substances that inhibit enzymes that can degrade cartilage. The chemical structure of chondroitin helps to create a watery, shock-absorbing space within cartilage tissue, resulting in better lubrication and nutrient transport in the joints. At the same time, chondroitin helps to attract fluid to the proteoglycan molecules. It also complements glucosamine as it boosts cartilage synthesis, inhibits the enzymes which destroy cartilage molecules, promotes cellular nourishment, and contributes to joint protection. French studies using oral chondroitin found that cartilage repair was significantly enhanced in patients using a three-month protocol of chondroitin.

METHYLSULFONYLMETHANE (MSM)

Methylsulfonylmethane (MSM) is a nutritional food supplement found in milk, fruits, meats and vegetables. Dr. Stanley Jacobs' clinical trials have demonstrated the safety and benefits of MSM as a source of organic sulfur. MSM has shown the remarkable ability to reduce muscle soreness, and cramps. It also helps alleviate the pain associated with systemic inflammatory disorders.

MELATONIN

In the 1950s scientists discovered melatonin, a hormone that may be the partial answer to sleep problems. It may also have the capability to affect other common distresses such as lack of immunity, aging, and cancer. Melatonin is produced by a small gland found in the center of the brain, the pineal gland. The pineal gland releases melatonin when the eye is not receiving light. Melatonin controls our sleep cycles and helps us to rest soundly. Another tremendous benefit of melatonin is that it contains vitamin E, one of the more powerful antioxidants and free radical fighters.

Administration of melatonin affects the three main characteristics of human sleep: 1) latency to sleep onset, 2) sleep consolidation "slow waves" and "sleep spindles," and 3) REM sleep (Dijk, 1997). It has been predicted that in the near future melatonin administration will become as useful as bright light exposure in the treatment of sleep disorders. The sleep-promoting effects of melatonin are typically observed within one hour following treatment, regardless of the time melatonin is administered (Zhdanova, 1997). For this reason it is advisable to restrict melatonin ingestion to the time just before retiring for the evening.

MALIC ACID

Malic acid is a food supplement found in citrus fruits and apples. Studies have found that it assists energy, metabolism, and production of muscle energy. When combined with magnesium, malic acid is a very powerful aid for the fibromyalgia sufferer. The citric acid cycle, sometimes called the tricarboxylic acid cycle or the Krebs cycle, is the main energy-producing cycle of the body. Malic acid enters the citric acid cycle at the most efficient site and is eventually converted into useable energy in the form of ATP (Lehninger, 1993).

A recent study shows the combined effects of malic acid and magnesium on fibromyalgia patients. Fifteen patients between the ages of 32 and 60 were used in an open clinical setting where oral magnesium and malic acid preparations were ingested for a period of four to eight weeks. The patients ingested 1200-2400 milligrams of malic acid with 30-600 milligrams of magnesium. The results of the study are encouraging as all patients reported significant relief of pain within just 48 hours of treatment. Results of studies such as this one gives us hope for the fibromyalgia patient through nutritional and supplemental treatment (Abraham, 1992).

PYCNOGENOL (PROANTHOCYANADINS)

Pycnogenol, a substance produced from grape seed extract and maritime pine bark, has been determined by scientists to be 50 times stronger than vitamin E. Its primary function is that of a very powerful antioxidant which scavenges free radicals generated by foreign toxic chemicals. It has also been thought to help remove inflammation from the joints and other tissues as well as improving the nervous and immune systems. Beyond that, pycnogenol strengthens collagen, improves circulation, enhances the permeability of cell walls, acts as a powerful antioxidant to boost the immune system, enhances metabolism, and promotes healing in the body. Human trials have shown that the flavonoids of pycnogenol can prevent peripheral hemorrhage, swelling of legs due to water retention, diabetic retinopathy, and high blood pressure (Lieberman, 1997).

RICE BRAN EXTRACT

Scientists have reportedly found that three of the tocotryonols in the polyphenols of rice bran carry a form of vitamin E that is 6,000 times stronger than the current forms of vitamin E. Vitamin E is a powerful antioxidant and helps with capillary wall strength, lung metabolism, muscle and nerve maintenance, and acts as an immune booster and detoxifier.

COENZYME Q10

The discovery of coenzyme Q10 is of tremendous benefit to mankind. It compares with vitamins A, C, and E as a powerful antioxidant. Research supports the fact that coenzyme Q10 benefits diseases associated with nutrient deficiencies such as cancer, aging, heart disease, obesity, and now fibromyalgia. This nutrient aids in the oxygenation of cells and tissues. It is found in food sources such as spinach, sardines, and peanuts. Coenzyme Q10 is estimated to be 20 times stronger than vitamin E and is considered to boost biochemical ability and activate cellular energy while improving circulation. One research study found that coenzyme Q10 literally doubled the immune system's ability to clear invading organisms from the blood.

DHEA (DEHYDROEPIANDOSTERONE)

DHEA, an adrenal hormone, is the most abundant hormone in the body and is often considered "the mother hormone." It is a precursor to the sex hormones as well as a number of other vital hormones in the body. Levels of DHEA are the highest when we are in the prime of life (age 20-35). DHEA is now available without prescription and has great value in preventing and treating osteoporosis, diabetes, cancer, Alzheimer's, cardiovascular disease, high cholesterol, and other immune disorders such as chronic fatigue syndrome and fibromyalgia. It is also thought to be effective in reducing the symptoms of PMS and menopause. It is sometimes called the "miracle" hormone because it is believed to slow down and even reverse the aging process. When recommended nutrients are ingested to boost and balance the bodily systems, then DHEA will be produced naturally and more readily in the body.

L-CARNITINE

L-carnitine is an amino acid that assists in breaking down fats and sugars for energy in the metabolic process. It is very effective with the fibromyalgia patient for raising energy levels.

CYSTEINE AND DERIVATIVES

Cysteine plays a critical role in the prevention of skeletal muscle wasting and fatigue conditions. The loss of body cell mass (wasting) is correlated with low baseline levels of plasma glutamine, arginine, and cystine. Wasting in healthy individuals appears to be self-terminating as glutamine, arginine, and cystine are adjusted to higher levels that stabilize body cell mass. Since cysteine and glutamine are related, the regulatory role of cysteine was tested in subjects with relatively low glutamine levels. Supplementation with N-acetyl-cysteine increased the ratio of body cell mass to body fat.

This indicates that cysteine does play a regulatory role in the maintenance of healthy body cell mass. In contrast, the placebo group showed a loss of body cell mass and an increase in body fat, suggesting that body protein had been converted into other forms of chemical energy. Low plasma glutamine in combination with high glutamate level risk for loss of body cell mass in healthy individuals: the effect of N-acetyl-cysteine (Kinscherf, 1996). The increased but unmet magnesium and cysteine requirements of fibromyalgia sufferers may explain the muscle pain they experience.

TRANSFER FACTOR

Our health and quality of life are directly influenced by our immune system. Today many factors contribute to the general weakening of our bodies' defenses. Antibiotics, commonly viewed as the most important advance in the history of medicine, have begun to fail as more and more microbes develop resistant strains. Fortunately, recent research has uncovered a natural agent—what are being called "transfer factor"—that can potentially save lives and increase the quality of life for many people.

Transfer factors are small immune messenger molecules that are produced by all higher organisms. They are both regulators of the immune system and carriers of the essential information needed by the immune system to identify foreign organisms. Transfer factor is unique to the infectious agent but are not dependent on the individual that produced them. Transfer factor produced by one person can be used in another person without concern for blood type or any other difference. In fact, transfer factors produced in animals and man are the same.

Colostrum, the first milk that a mother provides her offspring immediately after birth, is a rich source of transfer factor. This is nature's way of quickly educating a naive infant in the hazards of a microbe-infested world. One of the most abundant sources for transfer factor is found in the colostrum produced by cattle. Unfortunately, many people are allergic to milk proteins or are lactose-intolerant, making whole colostrum an unfit source of transfer factor for these persons. Recent technological breakthroughs have solved this problem. Transfer factor can now be efficiently isolated from bovine colostrum.

Transfer factor preparations have been used to educate the immune systems of persons suffering from chronic fatigue syndrome, a condition very similar to fibromyalgia. Like fibromyalgia, chronic fatigue syndrome is a syndrome with multiple contributing factors not the least of which is persistent viral infection. Because of the multiple infectious agents that can contribute to chronic fatigue syndrome, poly-valent (reactivity to more than one organism) transfer factor preparations have been used. Success was reported in 35 out of 39.

Another pilot study used poly-valent transfer factors with known potency for Epstein-Barr and Cytomegalovirus. In this study, two of the fourteen patients demonstrated total remission, while seven of the fourteen showed marked improvement. Use of a nonspecific transfer factor provided marked improvement in three out of six patients.

Immunological dysfunction is not the only contributing factor in fibromylagia but it is a critical issue that must be addressed. The involvement of viral infections in a large percentage of fibromyalgia cases has led researchers to propose viral infections as the initiating event for many fibromyalgia suffers. Overcoming the residual effects of viral damage and elimination of the persistent viral infections may be key in recovering from fibromyalgia.

PREGNENOLONE

Pregnenolone is one of the critical neurosteroids and has the ability to modify the sleep EEG in humans, which suggests its potential benefit as a memory enhancer (Baulieu, 1997). Studies conducted on acute shock stress indicate that there is a relationship between neurosteroid levels and the functional and emotional state of stressed animals (Parker, 1985). Such studies helped researchers to understand that a shift in the metabolism of pregnenolone may be necessary for survival during chronic severe stress. A very low dose of pregnenolone has been shown to significantly increase slow-wave, deep sleep in healthy human males. Neurosteroid pregnenolone induces sleep-EEG changes compatible with inverse agonist GABAA-receptor modulation (Steiger, 1993). Thus, it may be found that pregnenolone supplementation is beneficial to fibromyalgia patients.

GLUTAMINE AND UREA

Plasma cystine levels regulate nitrogen balance and body cell mass. The importance of maintaining normal cystine levels is so critical that skeletal muscle protein is cannibalized in order to supply the increased cystine demand. The role of cysteine and glutathione in HIV infection and other diseases is associated with muscle wasting and immunological disfunction (Droege, 1997). In the short term this may be useful, but in chronic conditions it is very damaging as it leads to an excess production of urea at the expense of glutamine that is needed for the fueling of the immune system.

CREATINE

A patent has been issued for the use of certain creatine preparations for treatment of fibromyalgia and other types of myopathy and cachectic states (Meyer 1998).

BEE POLLEN

Bee pollen is very high in protein and considered one of the most complete foods that we can consume. It contains vitamins, minerals, amino acids, proteins, enzymes, and fats. It helps when there is a hormone imbalance in the body. Bee pollen is very useful to fibromyalgia patients because it helps to increase appetite, normalize intestinal activity, strengthen capillary walls, offset the effects of drugs and pollutants, and is one of the most powerful immune boosters known to man.

GLUTATHIONE

The altered redox state in patients with rheumatoid arthritis indicate an important role for N-acetyl-L-cysteine (NAC) in the restoring of glutathione (GSH) levels in underactive joint T-cells. Such repletions of glutathione with NAC are well established.

References

Abraham, G., Russell, I.J., Michalek, J, and Flechas, J. "Treatment of Fibromyalgia syndrome with Super Malic: a randomized double blind, placebo controlled, crossover pilot study." *Journal of Rheumatology* 15, 22 (5), 53-8, 12

Baulieu, E.E. "Neurosteroids: of the nervous system, by the nervous system, for the nervous system." *Recent Prog Horm Res* 520, 1-32, 1997.

Bennett, R. M. "Beyond Fibromyalgia: Ideas on Etiology and Treatment," *Journal of Rheumatology* 16 (supple 19): 185, 1989.

Bucchi, L.H. 1995. *Pain Free*. Fort Worth, TX: The Summit Group.

Campbell, S. M., et al. "Clinical Characteristics of Fibrositis. I. A 'Blinded' Controlled Study of Symptoms and Tender Points," *Arthritis Rheumatology* 26: 817, 1983.

Clauw, D., Wilson B., Phadia S., Radulovic D., and Katz, K.P. "Low tissue levels of magnesium in fibromyalgia." *Clinical Research* 42(2), 141A, 1994.

Crofford, L. J. et al. "Hypothalamic-Pituitary-Adrenal Axis Perturbations in Patients with Fibromyalgia," *Arthritis Rheumatology* 37: 1583-1592, 1994.

Dijk, D.J.. "Melatonin and the circadian regulation of sleep 'initiation, consolidation, structure' and the sleep EEG." *Journal of Biology Rhythms* 12 (6), 627-35, 1997.

Droege,W., and Holm, E. *FASEB Journal* 11(13) 1077-1089, 1997.

Eisinger, J., Plantamura, A., Marie, P.A., and Ayavou T. "Selenium and magnesium in fibromyalgia." *Magnesium Research* 14, 7(3-4), 285-8, 1993.

Foster, Stephen. "Aloe Vera, easy to grow, easy to use." *Herbs for Health*. Jan/Feb 1997, 56.

Goldenberg, D. L. "Fibromyalgia and Chronic Fatigue Syndrome: Are They the Same?" *Journal of Musculoskeletal Medicine* 7: 19, 1990.

Kasper, S. *Pharmacopsychiatry* 30 (Suppl 20) 89-93, 1997.

Kinscherf, R., Hack, V., Fischbach, T., Friedmann, B., Weiss, C., Edler, L., Baertsch, P., and Droege, W. *Journal of Molecular Medicine* (Berlin) 74(7) 393-400, 1996.

Kitikar, K.R., and Basu, B.D. 1935. *Indian Medicinal Plants*, 521-9.

Laux, G. *Pharmacotherapy* (Ther Umsch) 54(10), 595-9, 1997.

Lehninger A.L., Nelson, D.L., and Cox, M.M. 1993. *Principles of Biochemistry*. New York: Worth Publishers.

Lieberman, S. Ph.D. and N. Bruning. 1997. *The Real Vitamin and Mineral Book*. Avery Publishing Group, 200.

Majeed, B., Badmaev, V., Gopinathan, S.R., Ajendran, R., and Norton, T. 1996. *Boswellian, the anti-iflammatory phytonutrient*. Piscataway, NJ: Nutriscience Publishers, Inc.

May, K. P. et al. "Sleep Apnea in Male Patients with the Fibromyalgia Syndrome," *American Journal of Medicine* 94:505,1993.

Meyer H, Wo 09800148, Ndn 172-0015-0324-7, 01-08-8.

Moldofsky, H. D. "Sleep, Neuroimmune and Neuroendocrine Functions in Fibromyalgia and Chronic Fatigue Syndrome," *Advances in Neuroimmunology* 5:39-56, 1995.

Mowrey, Daniel B. 1993. *Herbal Tonic Therapies*. New Canaan, CT: Keats

Publishing Inc., 152

Nicoldi, M., and Sicuteri, F. "Fibromyalgia and migraine, two faces of the same mechanism." *Adv Exp Med Biol.* 38, 73-9, 1996.

Null, Gary and Martin Feldman, M.D. 1993. *Reverse the Aging Process Naturally.* New York: Villard, 21.

Parker, L.N., Levin, E.R., and Lifrak, E.T., "Evidence for adrenocortical adaptation to severe illness." *J Clin Endocrin Metab* 60(5) 947-52, 1985.

Prudden, J.F., Migel, P., Hanson, P., Freidrich, L., and Balassa, L. "The discovery of a potent pure chemical wound-healing accelerator." *American Journal of Surgery* 119, 560, 1970.

Puttini, P.S. and Caruso, I. "Primary fibromyalgia syndrome and 5-hydroxyl-L-tryptophan: a 90-day open study." *J Int Med Res*, 20 (2), 182-9, 1996.

Sack, R.B. and Froelich, J.L. "Berberine inhibits intestinal secretory response of vibrio cholerae and *Escherichia coli* enterotizins." *Infectious Immunology*, 35, 471-475, 1982.

Singh, Y.N. "Kava: an overview. " *Journal of Ethnopharmacology* 37 (1), 13-45, 1992.

Steiger, A., Trachsel, L., Guldner, J., Hemmeter, U., Rothe, B., Rupprecht, R., Vedder, H., and Holsboer, F. *Brain Research* 615, 267-74, 1993.

Regland, B., Andersson, M., Abrahamsson, L., Babgby, J., Dyrehag, L.E., and Gottfries, C.G. "Increased concentrations of homocysteine in the cerebrospinal fluid inpatients with fibromyalgia and chronic fatigue syndrome." *Scandinavian Journal of Rheumatology* 26(4) 301-307, 1997.

Romano, T.J., and Stiller, J. "Magnesium deficiency in fibromyalgia syndrome." *Journal of Nutritional Medicine.* 14, 4(2) 165-67.

Russell, I. J. "Neurochemical Pathogenesis of Fibromyalgia Syndrome," *Journal of Musculoskeletal Pain* 4:61-92, 1996.

Weiner, Michael A. 1986. *Maximum Immunity.* Boston: Houghton Mifflin, 9.

Weintraub, S.

Wolfe, F. "Fibromyalgia: On Diagnosis and Certainty," *Journal of Musculoskeletal Pain* 1(3/4): 17, 1993.

Zhdanova, I.V. and Wurtman, R.J. "Efficacy of melatonin as a sleep-promoting agent." *Journal of Biological Rhythms*, 12(6) 588-4, 1997.